Sirtfood Diet Cookbook

The Power of Sirtuins Revealed:
Discover Scientifically Proven
Recipes to Burn Fat Fast

Ciaran Contreras

Dietado Publishing

Avocado egg boats

Prep time: 40min

Cook time: 8 minutes

Serves: 4

What you need:

- Freshly ground black pepper
- 2 ripe avocados, halved and pitted
- 3 slices bacon
- 4 large eggs Kosher salt
- Freshly chopped chives, for garnish

Method:

1. Firstly, preheat oven to 350°. Scoop about 1 tbsp. worth of avocado out of each half; discard or reserve for another use.
2. Put hollowed avocados in a baking dish, then crack eggs into a bowl, one at a time. Using a spoon, transfer one yolk to each avocado half, then spoon in as much egg white as you can fit without spilling over.
3. Add in salt and pepper and bake until whites are set and yolks are no longer runny, 20 to 25 minutes. (Cover with foil if avocados are beginning to brown.)
4. In the meantime, in a large skillet over medium heat, cook bacon until crisp, 8 minutes, then transfer to a paper towel-lined plate and chop.
5. Finally, top avocados with bacon and chives before serving.

Per serving: Calories 112 Fat 5g Protein 76g

Orzo risotto with cavolo Nero, peas and chili

Prep time: 30 min

Cook time: 12 minutes

Serves:2

What you need:

- extra-virgin olive oil 2 tsp
- garlic 2 cloves, sliced
- dried chili flakes ½ tsp
- vegetable stock 450ml, hot
- onion ½, finely diced
- orzo pasta 150g
- frozen peas 100g
- soft cheese 1 tablespoon
- cavolo Nero 100g, stems removed and cut into long pieces
- vegetarian parmesan 15g, finely grated, plus a little extra to serve (optional)

Method:

1. Firstly, heat the olive oil in a frying pan and add the onion, garlic, chili flakes and a pinch of salt. Cook gently for 5 minutes or until soft.
2. Toss in the pasta and stir so every piece is coated in oil. Add the vegetable stock a ladleful at a time, stirring in between and adding more once absorbed
3. After 5 minutes, add the cavolo Nero. Cook for a further 5 minutes and, once the orzo and cavolo Nero are tender, add the peas and some seasoning for a final 2 minutes.
4. Stir through the soft cheese and the parmesan, and serve with a little extra parmesan, if desired.

Per serving: Calories 221 Fat 6g Sugar 8g Protein 23g

Pomegranate guacamole

Prep time: 10 Minutes

Cook time: 40 Minutes

Serves:1

What you need:

- Flesh of 2 ripe avocados
- Seeds from 1 pomegranate
- 1 bird's-eye chili pepper, finely chopped
- ½ red onion, finely chopped
- Juice of 1 lime
- 151 calories per serving

Method:

1. Place the avocado, onion, chill and lime juice into a blender and process until smooth. Stir in the pomegranate seeds. Chill before serving. Serve as a dip for chop vegetables.

Per serving: Calories 151 Vitamin C 65g Fat 2 Protein 15

Tofu and curry

Prep time: 40 Minutes

Cook time: 10 Minutes

Serves:4

What you need:

- 8 oz. dried lentils red preferably
- 1 cup boiling water
- 1 cup frozen edamame soybeans
- 7 oz. 1/2 of most packages' firm tofu, chopped into cubes
- 2 tomatoes, chopped
- 1 lime juices
- 5-6 kale leaves, stalks removed and torn
- 1 large onion, chopped
- 4 cloves garlic, peeled and grated
- 1 large chunk of ginger, grated
- 1/2 red chili pepper, deseeded use less if too much
- 1/2 teaspoon ground turmeric
- 1/4 teaspoon cayenne pepper
- 1 teaspoon paprika
- 1/2 teaspoon ground cumin
- 1 teaspoon salt
- 1 tbsp. olive oil

Method:

1. Add the onion, sauté in the oil for few minutes then add the chili, garlic and ginger for a bit longer until wilted but not burned. Add the seasonings, then the lentils and stir. Add in the boiling water and cook for 10 minutes. Simmer for up to 30 minutes longer, so it will be stew-like but not overly mushy. You should check the texture of the lentils half way though.

2. Add tomato, tofu and edamame, then lime juice and kale. Test for when the kale is tender and then it is ready to serve.

Per serving: Calories 123 vitamin A 43g Fat 5 Proteins 43g

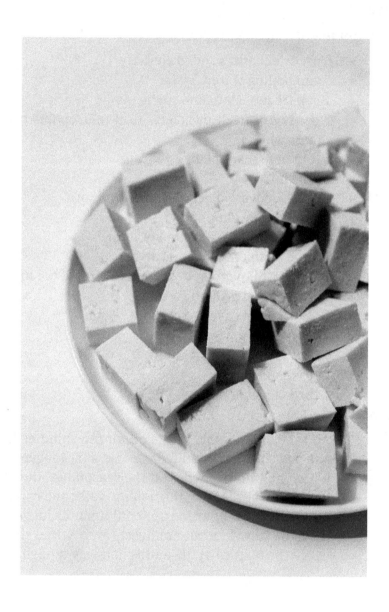

Garbanzo kale curry

Prep time:9 hours 30 Minutes

Cook time: 9 hours

Serves:8

What you need:

- 4 cups dry garbanzo beans
- Curry Paste, but go low on the heat
- 1 cup sliced tomato
- 2 cups kale leaves
- 1/2 cup coconut milk

Method:

1. Put ingredients in the slow cooker. Cover, & cook on low for 7 to 9 hours.

Per serving: Protein 98 Vitamin 54 Calories 95 Carbohydrates 103g

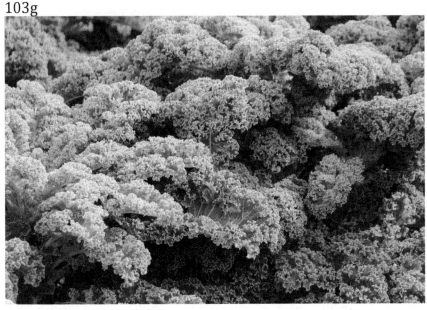

Miso-marinated baked cod with stir-fried greens and sesame

Prep time: 50 minutes

Cook time :20 minutes

Serves:1

What you need:

- 3 1/2 teaspoons (20g) miso
- 1 tablespoon mirin
- 1 tablespoon additional virgin olive oil
- 1 x 7-ounce (200g) skinless cod filet
- 1/8 cup (20g) red onion, cut
- 3/8 cup (40g) celery, cut
- 2 garlic cloves, finely hacked
- 1 Thai stew, finely cleaved
- 1 teaspoon finely hacked new ginger
- 3/8 cup (60g) green beans
- 3/4 cup (50g) kale, generally cleaved
- 1 teaspoon sesame seeds
- 2 tablespoons (5g) parsley, generally cleaved
- 1 tablespoon tamari (or soy sauce, if not evading gluten)
- 1/4 cup (40g) buckwheat
- 1 teaspoon ground turmeric

Method:

1. Blend the miso, mirin, and 1 teaspoon of the oil. Rub everywhere throughout the cod and leave to marinate for 30 minutes. Warmth the stove to 425oF (220oC).
2. Prepare the cod for 10 minutes.
3. In the interim, heat a huge skillet or wok with the rest of the oil. Include the onion and sautéed food for a couple of moments, at that point include the celery, garlic, stew, ginger, green beans, and kale. Hurl and

fry until the kale is delicate and cooked through. You may need to add a little water to the dish to help the cooking procedure.

4. Cook the buckwheat as indicated by the bundle directions along with the turmeric.
5. Include the sesame seeds, parsley, and tamari to the sautéed food and present with the buckwheat and fish.

Per serving: Calories 112 Fat 9g Protein 22g

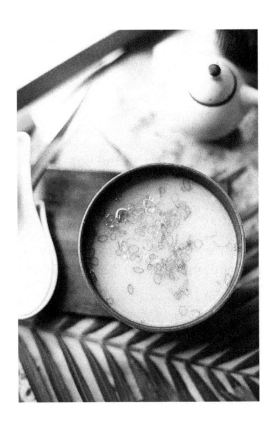

Poached eggs & rocket (arugula)

Prep time: 5 minutes

Cook time: 10 minutes

Serves: 4

What you need:

•2 eggs

•25g (1oz) fresh rocket (arugula)

•1 tsp olive oil

•sea salt

•freshly ground black pepper

Method:

1.Scatter the rocket (arugula) leaves onto a plate and drizzle the olive oil over them.

2.Bring a shallow pan of water to the boil, add in the eggs and cook until the whites become firm.

3.Serve the eggs on top of the rocket and season with salt and pepper.

Per serving: Calories 659, Calories from Fat 254, Total Fat 28.0g, Cholesterol 601mg, Sodium 3031mg, Total Carbohydrate 26.3g, Protein 75.7g.

Strawberry buckwheat pancakes

Prep time: 5 minutes

Cook time: 25 minutes

Serves: 4

What you need:

•100g (3½oz) strawberries, chopped

•100g (3½ oz) buckwheat flour

•1 egg

•250ml (8fl oz) milk

•1 tsp olive oil

•1 tsp olive oil for frying

•freshly squeezed juice of 1 orange

Method:

1.Pour the milk into a bowl and mix in the egg and a tsp of olive oil.

2.Sift in the flour to the liquid mixture until smooth and creamy.

3.Allow it to rest for 15 minutes.

4.Heat a little oil in a pan and pour in a quarter of the mixture (or to the size you prefer.)

5.Sprinkle in a quarter of the strawberries into the batter.

6.Cook for around 2 minutes on each side.

7.Serve hot with a drizzle of orange juice.

8.You could try experimenting with other berries such as blueberries and blackberries.

Per serving: Calories: 515 Carbs: 62.4g Protein: 9.3g Fats: 12. 8g

Snacks

No-Bake Blueberry Cheesecake Bars

Prep time: 15 minutes (not including crust)

Cook time: 7 minutes

Serves: 16

What you need:

- 2 (8-oz.) softened packages of Cream Cheese
- 1 Easy Shortbread Crust
- ¼ cup heavy whipping cream kept at room temp
- 1/2 cup of powdered Erythritol-based Sweetener
- 1 tsp grated Lemon Zest

Topping What you need:

- ¼ cup of Water
- 1 cup of Blueberries
- 1 tbsp fresh Lemon juice
- ¼ cup of powdered Erythritol-based Sweetener
- ¼ tsp Xanthan gum for garnish (optional)

Method:

Preparing the Bars:

1. Firmly press the crust mixture of the shortbread into the bottom of a baking pan. Place the crust in the refrigerator. Melt the chocolate in a bowl that you've set over a pan that placed on the water that just began simmering. Take the bowl out of the pan and allow it to cool for about 10 minutes.

2. With an electric mixer, beat the sweetener and the butter for 2 minutes until it is well incorporated and fluffy. Carefully add the melted chocolate while the mixer is running and continue beating until smooth. Add the salt, espresso powder, and vanilla extract. Add in the eggs one after the other and continue beating for 5 minutes. Carefully pour the filling ingredients on the top of the chilled crust and make sure to smoothen the top. Refrigerate for 2 hours.

Garnishing the Bars: Carefully spread the whipped cream and chocolate on top.

Per serving: Fat: 23.7g Carbs: 4.6g Protein: 4.6g Fiber: 2.2g Calories: 255

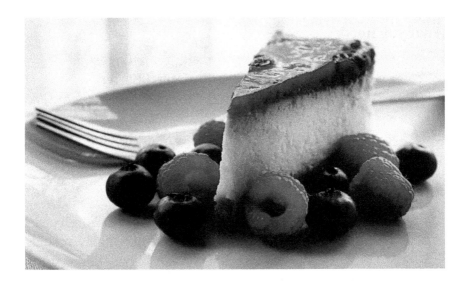

Chocolate-Covered Cheesecake Bites

Prep time: 20 minutes

Cook time: 5 minutes

Serves: 12

What you need:

- 1 (8 oz.) package of softened Cream Cheese
- ½ stick (¼ cup) unsalted softened Butter
- ½ cup of powdered Erythritol-based Sweetener
- ½ tsp. of vanilla extract
- 4 oz. of sugarless chopped Dark Chocolate
- 1½ tbsp. of Coconut oil or ¾ oz. of Cacao Butter

Method:

1. Line a baking sheet with parchment or wax paper.
2. Beat the butter and cream cheese with an electric mixer in a large bowl until it is thoroughly mixed. Beat in the vanilla extract and sweetener until smooth.
3. Form the mixture into 1-inch balls and position on the coated baking sheet.
4. Place them in the fridge for 3-4 hours until it becomes firm.
5. Melt the cacao butter and chocolate together over water that just began simmering over a heatproof bowl.
6. Stir until mixture becomes smooth. Remove from heat.
7. Dunk each ball into melted chocolate. Coat thoroughly and remove using a fork.
8. Firmly tap the fork on the sides of the bowl to eliminate extra chocolate.
9. Position the ball on the baking sheet and let it set.
10. Do the same for the rest of the cheesecake balls.
11. Decoratively sprinkle the rest of the chocolate over the lined balls.

Per serving: Fat: 13.5g Carbs: 5.2g Protein: 1.7g Fiber: 2.2g Calories: 148

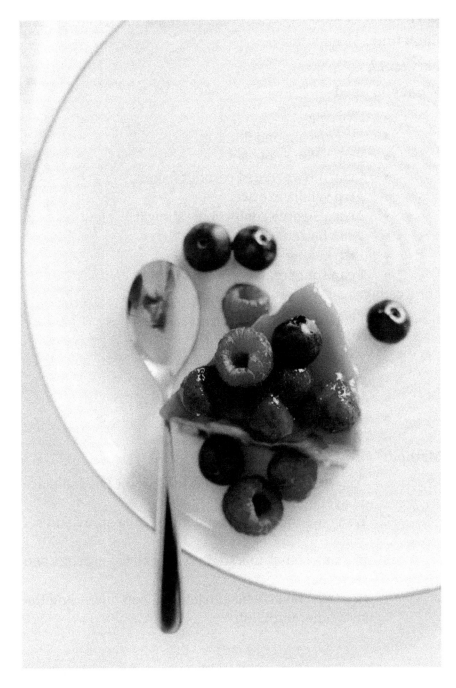

Delicious Italian Cake

Prep time: 10 minutes

Cook time: 55 minutes

Serves: 12

What you need:

- Five eggs
- 2½ cups almond flour
- 1 tsp baking powder
- 1 cup unsweetened coconut flakes
- 2 tsp vanilla extract
- 2 cups Swerve confectioners' sugar
- 1 cup butter
- 1 tsp baking soda
- 1 cup sour cream

For frosting:

- 1 cup unsweetened coconut flakes
- ½ cup walnuts, chopped
- 2 Tbsp unsweetened almond milk
- 2 cups Swerve confectioners' sugar
- 1 tsp vanilla extract
- ½ cup butter
- 8 oz cream cheese

Method:

1. Pour one cup of water into the Instant Pot and place a trivet in the pot.
2. Spray a 7-inch cake pan with cooking spray and set aside.
3. In a small bowl, mix sour cream and baking soda and set aside.
4. In a large bowl, whisk together 1 cup butter and the sweetener until fluffy.

5. Mix the eggs, almond flour, baking powder, 1 cup coconut flakes, 2 tsp vanilla, and the sour cream mixture.
6. Pour batter in the prepared cake pan—cover pan with aluminum foil.
7. Place the cake pan on top of the trivet in the Instant Pot.
8. Seal the pot with a lid and cook on manual mode for 35 minutes.
9. When finished, allow pressure to release naturally for 20 minutes, and then release using the quick release method. Open the lid.
10. Remove cake from the pot and let it cool completely.
11. For the frosting: In a mixing bowl, beat together ½ cup butter, Swerve, cream cheese, and vanilla until fluffy.
12. Add almond milk, walnuts, and coconut flakes and stir well.
13. Spread the frosting on top of the cake. Slice and serve.

Per serving: Calories 591 Fat 57.6 g Carbohydrates 11.3 g Protein 11.9 g

Tiramisu Sheet Cake

Prep time: 25 minutes

Cook time: 22 minutes

Serves: 20

What you need:

- ¾ cup granulated Erythritol-based Sweetener
- 0.44 lb. (2 cups) of blanched Almond flour
- 1/3 cup of unflavored Whey Protein powder
- 0.08 lb. (1/3 cup) of Coconut flour
- 1 tbsp. of baking Powder
- 1/2 tsp. of salt
- One stick (½ cup) of unsalted and melted butter
- ¾ cup of unsweetened Almond Milk
- One tsp. of Vanilla extract
- Three large eggs
- One tbs. of dark Rum (optional)
- ¼ cup of cooled strong brewed coffee or espresso
- Mascarpone Frosting What you need:
- 4 oz. (½ cup) of softened Cream Cheese
- 8 oz. of softened Mascarpone Cheese
- One tsp. of Vanilla extract
- A ½-2/3 cup of heavy Whipping cream kept at room temp
- ½ cup of powdered Erythritol-based Sweetener
- Ingredients for Garnishing:
- 1-oz. of sugarless dark Chocolate
- 1 tbsp. of Cocoa powder

Method:

1. In a blender or food processor, grind the macadamia nuts to a beautiful texture.
2. Add all the cinnamon roll ingredients except for caramel sauce, and then put in the refrigerator to chill for an hour.

3. Heat the oven to 350° F. Line a baking tray with parchment paper.
4. Roll out the dough and make a large rectangle shape on a parchment-lined surface.
5. Spread the Keto Caramel Sauce over the batter.
6. Carefully roll the dough into a log shape and seal the edge.
7. Place a sharp knife in warm water and cut the log into about 10-12 rolls.
8. Position rolls on coated tray and place in the oven for 25 to 30 minutes, making sure that you check after 20 minutes to check if it cooked through.
9. While the cinnamon rolls are baking in the oven, make the glaze. Combine all ingredients in a blender or mixing bowl.
10. Take keto cinnamon rolls out of the oven. Let it cool before you glaze. You can serve warm with glaze garnished on the top.

Per serving: Calories: 477 Fat: 45.6g Carbs: 17.1g Fiber: 7.1g Protein: 5.6g

Cinnamon Crumb Cake Keto Donuts

Prep time: 10 minutes

Cook time: 15 minutes

Serves: 1

What you need:

- ½ cup of Coconut flour
- ¼ cup of Almond flour
- 1 tbsp of Flaxseed meal
- 1 tsp of baking powder
- ¼ tsp salt
- 1 tsp of Cinnamon
- ¼ tsp of Nutmeg
- 2/3 cup of Erythritol Sweetener (e.g. Swerve)
- Six large eggs
- ½ cup of butter, melted
- 1 tsp of vanilla
- ½ cup of Almond flour
- ¼ cup of diced pecans (optional)
- One pinch of salt
- 2 tbsp of softened butter

Method:

1. Heat the oven to 350° F.
2. Use a non-stick spray to spray a doughnut pan.
3. Preparing the doughnuts:
4. Whisk the coconut flour, almond flour, flax meal, sweetener, baking powder, salt, nutmeg, and Cinnamon together inside a medium bowl. Set aside.
5. Whisk the eggs, vanilla, and melted butter until it appears. Add all the dry ingredients into wet ingredients and mix.
6. Spoon the batter into the doughnut space and fill it ¾ of the way full.
7. Preparing the crumb topping:

8. Stir together the sweetener, almond meal, and salt inside a small bowl. Add the butter and mix. Thoroughly mix until all of the flour is well combined, and the mixture moistened.
9. Topping the doughnuts:
10. Garnish the topping on the doughnuts, with fingers to break up the mixture until it is well mixed.
11. Place in the oven for 12-15 minutes or until the sides appear light brown.

Per serving: Calories: 138g Fat: 12g Carbs: 3g Fiber: 2g Protein: 4g

Espresso Chocolate Cheesecake Bars

Prep time: 10 minutes

Cook time: 35 minutes

Serves: 16

What you need:

- 7 tbsp. of melted Butter
- 2 cups of ultrafine, blanched Almond flour
- 3 tbsp. of Cocoa powder
- 1/3 cup granulated Erythritol sweetener
- Cheesecake What you need:
- 16 oz. of full fat Cream Cheese
- Two large eggs
- ½ cup of granulated Erythritol sweetener
- 2 tbsp. of instant Espresso powder
- One tsp. of Vanilla extract
- Extra cocoa powder for dusting over the top.

Method:

1. Preparation of the Chocolate Crust:
2. Heat the oven to 350° F.
3. Combine the almond flour, melted butter, cocoa powder, and sweetener in a medium-sized bowl.
4. Transfer the crust dough to a 9 x 9" pan coated with foil or parchment paper.
5. Firmly press the crust to the bottom of the pan.
6. Place the crust in the oven and bake for about 8 minutes.
7. Take out of the oven and set aside to cool.
8. Preparing the cheesecake filling:
9. Place the eggs, cream cheese, espresso powder, vanilla extract, and sweetener inside a blender and blend the mixture until smooth.
10. Pour over the crust and evenly spread out in the pan.
11. Bake for 25 minutes. Take out of the oven and allow it to cool. Dust it with the cocoa powder

12. Place in the refrigerator to chill. Afterwards, cut into four rows of squares to serve.

Per serving: Calories: 232 Fat: 21g Carbs: 5g Fiber: 1.5g Protein: 6g

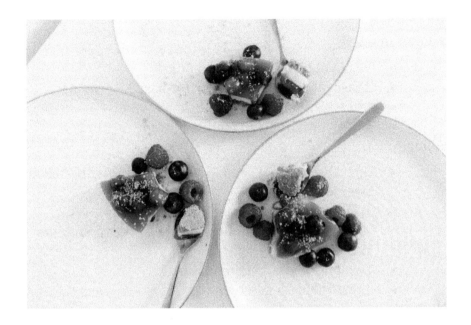

Mini No-Bake Lemon Cheesecakes

Prep time: 20 minutes

Cook time: 0

Serves: 6

What you need:

- ½ cup of blanched almond flour
- 2 tbsp. of powdered Erythritol-based Sweetener
- 1/8 tsp. of salt
- 2 tbsp. unsalted and melted butter

Filling:

- One tbs. plus ¼ cup powdered Erythritol-based Sweetener
- ¾ cup (6 oz.) of softened Cream Cheese
- ¼ cup of heavy whipping cream kept at room temp
- ½ tsp. of Lemon extract
- Two tsp. of grated Lemon Zest
- 2 tbsp. of fresh Lemon juice

Method:

1. Preparing the Crust What you need:
2. Line muffin pan with parchment paper or silicone.
3. Whisk the sweetener, almond flour. Add the melted butter and stir until mixture starts clumping together.
4. Place the crust in the muffin cups you've prepared and made sure to press into the bottoms firmly.
5. Preparing the Filling:
6. With an electric mixer, beat the cream cheese in a medium bowl. Add the sweetener until it is well combined.
7. Beat in the lemon extract, lemon juice, lemon zest, and the cream until smooth.
8. Share the filling mixture into the muffin cups you prepared and fill all of the containers to almost the

top. Also, smoothen the top. To let go of air bubbles firmly tap the pan on a counter.

9. For 2 hours, place the pan in the fridge so that the filling becomes firm. Carefully remove the silicone layers or the parchment paper liners. Serve when ready.

Per serving: Fat: 20.1g Carbs: 3.9g Protein: 4g Fiber: 1.1g Calories: 223

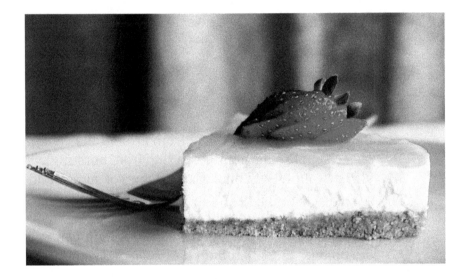

Baked Maple Apple

Prep time: 10 minutes

Cook time: 30 minutes

Serves: 2

What you need:

- Two small apples
- Two teaspoons reduced-calorie apricot
- spread (16 calories per 2teaspoons)
- One teaspoon reduced-calorie maple-flavored syrup (60 calories per fluid ounce)

Method:

1. Remove the core from each apple to 1/2 inch from the bottom.
2. Remove a thin strip of peel from around the center of each apple (this helps keep skin from bursting).
3. Fill each apple with one teaspoon apricot spread and 1/2 teaspoon maple syrup.
4. Place each apple upright in individual baking dish; cover dishes with foil and bake at 400°F until apples are tender, 25 to 30 minutes.

Per serving: 75 calories. 0.2 g protein. 1 g fat. 19 g carbohydrate. 0.3 mg sodium. 0 mg cholesterol

Apple-Raisin Cake

Prep time: 10 minutes

Cook time: 50 minutes

Serves: 12

What you need:

- One teaspoon baking soda
- 1/2 cups applesauce (no sugar added)
- Two small Golden Delicious apples, cored, pared, and shredded
- 1 cup less 2 tablespoons raisins
- 2/4 cups self-rising flour
- 1 teaspoon ground cinnamon
- 1/2 teaspoon ground cloves 1/3 cup plus 2 teaspoons unsalted margarine
- 1/4 cup granulated sugar

Method:

1. Spray an 8 x 8 x 2-inch baking pan with nonstick cooking spray and set aside. Into a medium bowl sift together flour, cinnamon, and cloves; set aside.
2. Preheat oven to 350°F. In a medium mixing bowl, using an electric mixer, cream margarine, add sugar and stir to combine.
3. Stir baking soda into applesauce, then add to margarine mixture and stir to combine; add sifted ingredients and, using an electric mixer on medium speed, beat until thoroughly combined.
4. Fold in apples and raisins; pour batter into the sprayed pan and bake for 45 to 50 minutes (until cake is browned and a cake tester or toothpick, inserted in center, comes out dry).
5. Remove cake from pan and cool on wire rack.

Per serving: 151 calories. 2 g protein.4 g fat. 28 g carbohydrate. 96 mg sodium. 0 mg cholesterol

Cinnamon-Apricot Bananas

Prep time: 10 minutes

Cook time: 20 minutes

Serves: 2

What you need:

- 4 graham crackers 2x2-inch 1 medium banana, peeled and cut in squares), made into crumbs half lengthwise
- 2 teaspoons shredded coconut
- 1/4 teaspoon ground cinnamon
- 1 tablespoon plus 1 teaspoon reduced-calorie apricot spread (16 calories per 2 teaspoons)

Method:

1. In small skillet combine crumbs, coconut, and cinnamon and toast lightly, being careful not to burn; transfer to a sheet of wax paper or a paper plate and set aside.
2. In the same skillet heat apricot spread until melted; remove from heat. Roll each banana half in a spread, then quickly roll in crumb mixture, pressing crumbs so that they adhere to the banana; place coated halves on a plate, cover lightly, and refrigerate until chilled.
3. Variation: Coconut-Strawberry Bananas —Omit cinnamon and substitute reduced-calorie strawberry spread (16 calories per 2 teaspoons) for the apricot spread.

Per serving: 130 calories.2 g protein. 2 g fat. 29 g carbohydrate. 95 mg sodium.0 mg cholesterol

Meringue Crepes with Blueberry Custard Filling

Prep time: 10 minutes

Cook time: 20 minutes

Serves: 4

What you need:

- 2 cups blueberries (reserve 8 berries for garnish)
- 8 crepes
- 1 cup evaporated skimmed milk
- 2 large eggs, separated
- 1 tablespoon plus 1 teaspoon
- granulated sugar, divided
- 2 teaspoons each cornstarch
- lemon juice

Method:

1. In 1-quart saucepan, combine milk, egg yolks, and one tablespoon sugar; cook over low heat, continually stirring, until slightly thickened and bubbles form around sides of the mixture. In a cup or small bowl dissolve cornstarch in lemon juice; gradually stir into milk mixture and cook, constantly stirring, until thick. Remove from heat and fold in blueberries; let cool.
2. Spoon Vs. of custard onto the center of each crepe and fold sides over filling to enclose; arrange crepes, seam-side down, in an 8 x 8 x 2-inch baking pan. In a small bowl, using an electric mixer on high speed, beat egg whites until soft peaks form; add remaining teaspoon sugar, and continue beating until stiff peaks form.
3. Fill the pastry bag with egg whites and pipe an equal amount over each crepe (if pastry bag is not available, spoon egg whites over crepes); top each

with a reserved blueberry and broil until meringue is lightly browned, 10 to 15 seconds. Serve immediately.

Per serving: 300 calories.16 g protein. 6 g fat. 45 g carbohydrate. 180 mg sodium. 278 mg cholesterol

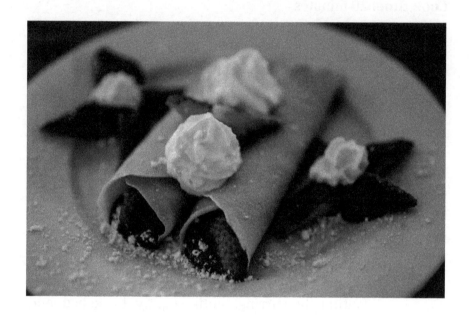

Meatless Borscht

Prep time: 10 minutes

Cook time: 25 minutes

Serves: 2

What you need:

- 1 teaspoon margarine
- 1 cup shredded green cabbage
- 1/4 cup chopped onion
- 1/4 cup sliced carrot
- 1 cup coarsely shredded pared
- 2 tablespoons tomato paste beets
- 1 tablespoon lemon juice
- 2 cups of water
- 1/2 teaspoon granulated sugar
- 2 packets instant beef broth and 1 teaspoon pepper
- seasoning mix
- 1/4 cup plain low-fat yogurt
- 1/2 bay leaf

Method:

1. In 1 1/2-quart saucepan heat margarine until bubbly and hot; add onion and sauté until softened, 1 to 2 minutes.
2. Add beets and toss to combine; add water, broth mix, and bay leaf and bring to a boil.
3. Cover pan and cook over medium heat for 10 minutes; stir in remaining ingredients except for yogurt, cover, and let simmer until vegetables are tender about 25 minutes.
4. Remove and discard bay leaf. Pour borscht into 2 soup bowls and top each portion with 2 tablespoons yogurt.

Per serving: 120 calories. 5 g protein. 3 g fat. 21 g carbohydrate. 982 mg sodium. 2 mg cholesterol

Sauteed Sweet 'n' Sour Beets

Prep time: 5 minutes

Cook time: 10 minutes

Serves: 2

What you need:

- 2 teaspoons margarine
- 1 tablespoon diced onion
- 1 cup drained canned small whole beets, cut into quarters
- 1 tablespoon each lemon juice and water
- 1 teaspoon each salt and pepper
- Dash granulated sugar substitute

Method:

1. In small nonstick skillet heat margarine over medium-high heat until bubbly and hot; add onion and sauté until softened, 1 to 2 minutes.
2. Reduce heat to low and add remaining ingredients; cover pan and cook, stirring once, for 5 minutes longer.

Per serving: 70 calories. 1 g protein. 4 g fat. 9 g carbohydrate. 385 mg sodium. 0 mg cholesterol

Orange Beets

Prep time: 5 minutes

Cook time: 20 minutes

Serves: 2

- **What you need:**
- 1 /2 teaspoons lemon juice
- 1 teaspoon cornstarch Dash salt
- 1 teaspoon orange marmalade
- 1 cup peeled and sliced cooked beets
- 2 teaspoons margarine
- 1 teaspoon firmly packed brown
- sugar 1/4 cup orange juice (no sugar added)

Method:

1. In a 1-quart saucepan (not aluminum or cast-iron), combine beets, margarine, and sugar; cook over low heat, continually stirring until margarine and sugar are melted.
2. In 1-cup measure or small bowl combine juices, cornstarch, and salt, stirring to dissolve cornstarch; pour over beet mixture and, constantly stirring, bring to a boil. Continue cooking and stirring until the mixture thickens.
3. Reduce heat, add marmalade, and stir until combined. Remove from heat and let cool slightly; cover and refrigerate for at least 1 hour. Reheat before serving.

Per serving: 99 calories. 1 g protein. 4 g fat.16 g carbohydrate. 146 mg sodium. 0 mg cholesterol

Cabbage 'n' Potato Soup

Prep time: 10 minutes

Cook time: 30 minutes

Serves: 4

What you need:

- 2 teaspoons vegetable oil
- 4 cups shredded green cabbage
- 1 cup sliced onions
- 1 garlic clove, minced
- 3 cups of water
- 6 ounces peeled potato, sliced
- 1 cup each sliced carrot and tomato puree
- 4 packets instant beef broth and seasoning mix
- 1 each bay leaf and whole clove

Method:

1. In 2-quart saucepan heat oil, add cabbage, onions, and garlic and sauté over medium heat, frequently stirring, until cabbage is soft, about 10 minutes.
2. Reduce heat to low and add remaining ingredients; cook until vegetables are tender, about 30 minutes.
3. Remove and discard bay leaf and clove before serving.

Per serving: 119 calories.4 g protein. 3 g fat.22 g carbohydrate. 900 mg sodium, 0 mg cholesterol.

Spicy Ras-el-Hanout Dressing

Prep time:10 minutes

Cook time:0 minutes

Serves:1

Ingredients

- 125ml Olive oil
- 1-piece Lemon (the juice)
- 2teaspoons Honey
- 1 ½teaspoons Ras el Hanout
- ½ pieces Red pepper

Method:

1. Remove the seeds from the chili pepper.
2. Chop the chili pepper as finely as possible.
3. Place the pepper in a bowl with lemon juice, honey, and Ras-El-Hanout and whisk with a whisk.
4. Then add the olive oil drop by drop while continuing to whisk.

Per serving: Energy (calories): 81 kcal; Protein: 1.32 g; Fat: 0.86 g; Carbohydrates: 20.02 g

Chicken Rolls with Pesto

Prep time: 10 minutes

Cook time: 10 minutes

Serves: 2

What you need:

- 2tablespoon Pine nuts
- 25g Yeast flakes
- 1clove Garlic (chopped)
- 15g fresh basil
- 85ml Olive oil
- 2pieces Chicken breast

Method:

1. Preheat the oven to 175 ° C.
2. Roast the pine nuts in a dry pan over medium heat for 3 minutes until golden brown. Place on a plate and set aside.
3. Put the pine nuts, yeast flakes and garlic in a food processor and grind them finely.
4. Add the basil and oil and mix briefly until you get a pesto.
5. Season with salt and pepper.
6. Place each piece of chicken breast between 2 pieces of cling film
7. Beat with a saucepan or rolling pin until the chicken breast is about 0.6 cm thick.
8. Remove the cling film and spread the pesto on the chicken.
9. Roll up the chicken breasts and use cocktail skewers to hold them together.

Per serving: Energy (calories): 527 kcal; Protein: 63.8 g; Fat: 27.1 g; Carbohydrates: 3.27 g

Mustard

Prep time: 10 minutes

Cook time:0 minutes

Serves:1

What you need:

- 60g Mustard seeds
- 60ml Water
- 60ml Apple cider vinegar
- 2teaspoons Lemon juice
- 90g Honey
- ½ teaspoon dried turmeric

Method:

1. Put mustard seeds, water and vinegar in a glass, close well and leave in the fridge for 12 hours.
2. Put all ingredients in a tall measuring cup the next day.
3. Use your hand blender to puree everything.
4. Try the mustard and add some honey or salt.
5. Store the mustard in a clean glass in the fridge, it will keep for at least 3 weeks.

Per serving: Energy (calories): 590 kcal; Protein: 16.24 g; Fat: 21.87 g; Carbohydrates: 93.73 g

Vegetarian Curry from The Crock Pot

Prep time:20 minutes

Cook time:6 hours

Serves:1

What you need:

- 4pieces Carrot
- 2pieces Sweet potato
- 1-piece Onion
- 3cloves Garlic
- 2tablespoon Curry powder
- 1teaspoon Ground caraway (ground)
- ¼ teaspoon Chili powder
- 1/4 TL Celtic sea salt
- 1pinch Cinnamon
- 100ml Vegetable broth
- 400g Tomato cubes (can)
- 250g Sweet peas
- 2tablespoon Tapioca flour

Method:

1. Roughly chop vegetables and potatoes and press garlic. Halve the sugar snap peas.
2. Put the carrots, sweet potatoes and onions in the slow cooker.
3. Mix tapioca flour with curry powder, cumin, chili powder, salt and cinnamon and sprinkle this mixture on the vegetables.
4. Pour the vegetable broth over it.
5. Close the lid of the slow cooker and let it simmer for 6 hours on a low setting.
6. Stir in the tomatoes and sugar snap peas for the last hour.

Per serving: Energy (calories): 794 kcal; Protein: 18.7 g; Fat: 12.14 g; Carbohydrates: 163.11 g

Fried Cauliflower Rice

Prep time:10 minutes

Cook time:10 minutes

Serves:1

Ingredients

- 1-piece Cauliflower
- 2 tablespoon Coconut oil
- 1-piece Red onion
- 4cloves Garlic
- 60ml Vegetable broth
- 1.5cm fresh ginger
- 1 teaspoon Chili flakes
- ½ pieces Carrot
- ½ pieces Red bell pepper
- ½ pieces Lemon (the juice)
- 2 tablespoon Pumpkin seeds
- 2 tablespoon fresh coriander

Method:

1. Cut the cauliflower into small rice grains in a food processor.
2. Finely chop the onion, garlic and ginger, cut the carrot into thin strips, dice the bell pepper and finely chop the herbs.
3. Melt 1 tablespoon of coconut oil in a pan and add half of the onion and garlic to the pan and fry briefly until translucent.
4. Add cauliflower rice and season with salt.
5. Pour in the broth and stir everything until it evaporates and the cauliflower rice is tender. Take the rice out of the pan and set it aside.
6. Melt the rest of the coconut oil in the pan and add the remaining onions, garlic, ginger, carrots and peppers.

7. Fry for a few minutes until the vegetables are tender. Season them with a little salt.
8. Add the cauliflower rice again, heat the whole dish and add the lemon juice.

Per serving: Energy (calories): 461 kcal; Protein: 10.27 g; Fat: 35.61 g; Carbohydrates: 34.5 g

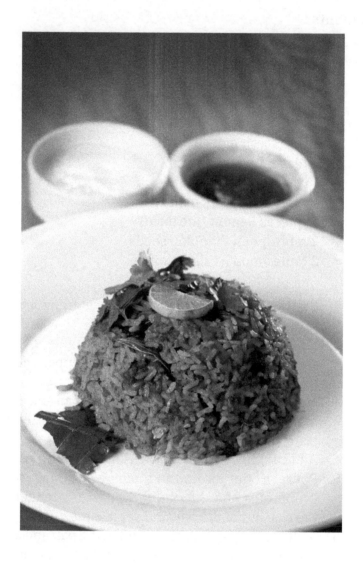

Pizza

Prep time: 10 minutes

Cook time: 10 minutes

Serves: 2

What you need:

For the pizza crusts:

- 120g Tapioca flour
- 1 teaspoon Celtic sea salt
- 2 tablespoon Italian spice mix
- 45g Coconut flour
- 120ml Olive oil (mild)
- Water (warm) 120 ml
- Egg (beaten) 1 piece

For covering:

- 2tablespoon Tomato paste
- ½ pieces Zucchini
- ½ pieces Eggplant
- 2 pieces Tomato
- 2 tablespoon Olive oil (mild)
- 1 tablespoon Balsamic vinegar

Method:

1. Preheat the oven to 190 ° C and line a baking sheet with parchment paper.
2. Cut the vegetables into thin slices.
3. Mix the tapioca flour with salt, Italian herbs and coconut flour in a large bowl.
4. Pour in olive oil and warm water and stir well.
5. Then add the egg and stir until you get an even dough.
6. If the dough is thin, add 1 tablespoon of coconut flour at a time until it is the desired thickness. Always wait a few minutes before adding more coconut flour, as

it will take some time to absorb the moisture. The intent is to get a soft, sticky dough.

7. Divide the dough into two parts and spread them in flat circles on the baking sheet (or make 1 large sheet of pizza as shown in the picture).
8. Bake in the oven for about 10 minutes.
9. Brush the pizza with tomato paste and spread the Aubergine, zucchini and tomato overlapping on the pizza.

Per serving: Energy (calories): 514 kcal; Protein: 9.64 g; Fat: 19.32 g; Carbohydrates: 79.22 g

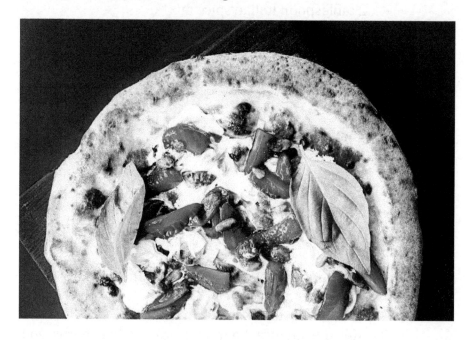

Vegetarian Paleo Ratatouille

Prep time: 0 minutes

Cook time: 0 minutes

Serves: 1

What you need:

- 200g Tomato cubes (can)
- ½ pieces Onion
- 2cloves Garlic
- ¼ teaspoon dried oregano
- 1 / 4TL Chili flakes
- 2tablespoon Olive oil
- 1Piece Eggplant
- 1Piece Zucchini
- 1Piece hot peppers
- 1teaspoon dried thyme

Method:

1. Preheat the oven to 180 ° C and lightly grease a round or oval shape.
2. Finely chop the onion and garlic.
3. Mix the tomato cubes with garlic, onion, oregano and chili flakes, season with salt and pepper and put on the bottom of the baking dish.
4. Use a mandolin, a cheese slicer or a sharp knife to cut the eggplant, zucchini and hot pepper into very thin slices.
5. Put the vegetables in a bowl (make circles, start at the edge and work inside).
6. Drizzle the remaining olive oil on the vegetables and sprinkle with thyme, salt and pepper.
7. Cover the baking dish with a piece of parchment paper and bake in the oven for 45 to 55 minutes.

Per serving: Energy (calories): 546 kcal; Protein: 11.31 g; Fat: 28.97 g; Carbohydrates: 71.62 g

Courgette and Broccoli Soup:

Prep time: 10 minutes

Cook time: 55 minutes

Serves: 1

What you need:

- 2tablespoon Coconut oil
- 1Piece Red onion
- 2Cloves Garlic
- 300g Broccoli
- 1Piece Zucchini
- 750ml Vegetable broth

Method:

1. Finely chop the onion and garlic, cut the broccoli into florets and the zucchini into slices.
2. Melt the coconut oil in a soup pot and fry the onion with the garlic.
3. Cook the zucchini for a few minutes.
4. Add broccoli and vegetable broth and simmer for about 5 minutes.
5. Puree the soup with a hand blender and season with salt and pepper.

Per serving: Energy (calories): 342 kcal; Protein: 18.12 g; Fat: 23.48 g; Carbohydrates: 35.27 g

Frittata with Spring Onions and Asparagus

Prep time: 10 minutes

Cook time: 30 minutes

Serves: 1

What you need:

- 5pieces Egg
- 80ml Almond milk
- 2tablespoon Coconut oil
- 1clove Garlic
- 100g Asparagus tips
- 4pieces Spring onions
- 1teaspoon Tarragon
- 1pinch Chili flakes

Method:

1. Preheat the oven to 220 ° C.
2. Squeeze the garlic and finely chop the spring onions.
3. Whisk the eggs with the almond milk and season with salt and pepper.
4. Melt 1 tablespoon of coconut oil in a medium-sized cast iron pan and briefly fry the onion and garlic with the asparagus.
5. Remove the vegetables from the pan and melt the remaining coconut oil in the pan.
6. Pour in the egg mixture and half of the entire vegetable.
7. Place the pan in the oven for 15 minutes until the egg has solidified.
8. Then take the pan out of the oven and pour the rest of the egg with the vegetables into the pan.
9. Place the pan in the oven again for 15 minutes until the egg is nice and loose.
10. Sprinkle the tarragon and chili flakes on the dish before serving.

Per serving: Energy (calories): 464 kcal; Protein: 24.23 g; Fat: 37.84 g; Carbohydrates: 7.33 g

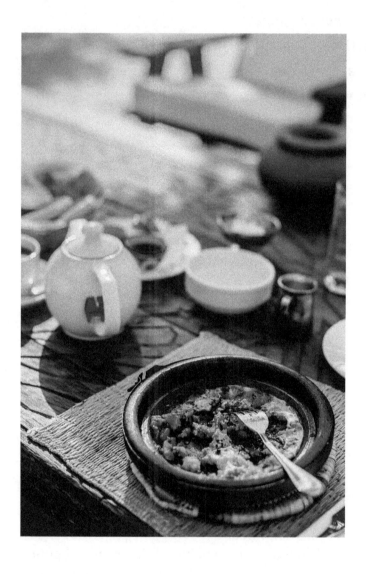

Cucumber Salad with Lime and Coriander

Prep time: 10 minutes

Cook time: 0 minutes

Serves: 1

What you need:

- 1Piece Red onion
- 2Pieces Cucumber
- 2Pieces Lime (juice)
- 2Tablespoon fresh coriander

Method:

1. Cut the onion into rings and thinly slice the cucumber. Chop the coriander finely.
2. Place the onion rings in a bowl and season with about half a tablespoon of salt.
3. Rub it in well and then fill the bowl with water.
4. Pour off the water and then rinse the onion rings thoroughly (in a sieve).
5. Put the cucumber slices together with onion, lime juice, coriander and olive oil in a salad bowl and stir everything well.

Per serving: Energy (calories): 115 kcal; Protein: 3.99 g; Fat: 0.83 g; Carbohydrates: 26.44 g

. Home-Made Marshmallow Fluff

Prep time:10 minutes

Cook time:10 minutes

Serves:10

What you need:

- 3/4cup sugar
- 1/2cup light corn syrup
- 1/4cup water
- 1/8 tsp salt
- 3little egg whites

- 1/4tsp cream of tartar
- 1teaspoon 1/2 tsp vanilla extract

Method:

1. In a little pan, mix together sugar, corn syrup, salt and water. Attach a candy thermometer into the side of this pan, but make sure it will not touch the underside of the pan.
2. From the bowl of a stand mixer, combine egg whites and cream of tartar. Begin to whip on medium speed with the whisk attachment.
3. Meanwhile, turn a burner on top and place the pan with the sugar mix onto heat. Pout mix into a boil and heat to 240 degrees, stirring periodically.
4. The aim is to have the egg whites whipped to soft peaks and also the sugar heated to 240 degrees at near the same moment. Simply stop stirring the egg whites once they hit soft peaks.
5. Once the sugar has already reached 240 amounts, turn heat low allowing it to reduce. Insert a little quantity of the popular sugar mix and let it mix. Insert still another little sum of the sugar mix. Add mix slowly and that means you never scramble the egg whites.
6. After all of the sugar was added into the egg whites, then decrease the speed of the mixer and also keep mixing concoction for around 7- 9 minutes until the fluff remains glossy and stiff. At roughly the 5-minute mark, then add the vanilla extract.

Per serving: Energy (calories): 84 kcal; Protein: 1.08 g; Fat: 0.08 g; Carbohydrates: 20.71 g

Berry Smoothie

Prep time: 5 Minutes

Cook time: 1 Minute

Serves: 1

What you need:

- Two scoops Protein Powder 2 cups Almond Milk
- 4 cups Mixed Berry
- 2 cups Yoghurt

Method:

1. First, place mixed berry, protein powder, yoghurt, and almond milk in the blender pitcher.
2. Then, select the 'smoothie' button.
3. Finally, pour the smoothie to the serving glass. To make it more nutritious and filling, you can even add banana to it.

Per serving: Calories: 306 •Carbs: 36g •Fat: 3g •Protein: 36g. 306.

Avocado Smoothie

Prep time: 5 Minutes

Cook time: 5 Minutes

Serves: 2

What you need:

- 1 cup Coconut Milk, preferably full-fat
- 1 cup Ice
- 3 cups Baby Spinach
- 1 Banana, frozen & quartered
- 1/2 cup pineapple chunks, frozen
- 1/2 of 1 Avocado, smooth

Method:

1. First, place ice, pineapple chunks, pineapple chunks, banana, avocado, baby spinach in the blender pitcher.
2. Now, press the 'extract' button.
3. Finally, transfer to a serving glass.
4. To make it more nutritious and filling, you can even add banana to it.

Per serving: Calories 236, Protein 8g, Carbohydrate 46g, Fat 10g.

Tofu Smoothie

Prep time: 5 Minutes

Cook time: 5 Minutes

Serves: 2

What you need:

- 1 Banana, sliced & frozen
- 3/4 cup Almond Milk
- 2 tbsp. Peanut Butter
- 1/2 cup Yoghurt, plain & low-fat
- 1/2 cup Tofu, soft & silken
- 1/3 cup Dates, chopped

Method:

1. First, place tofu, banana, dates, yogurt, peanut butter, and almond milk in the blender pitcher.
2. After that, press the 'smoothie' button.
3. Finally, transfer to serving glass and enjoy it.

Tip: You can try adding herbs to your preference.

Per serving: Calories: 119 Sugar: 13 Sodium: 31 Fat: 2 Carbohydrates: 22 Fiber: 3 Protein: 5

Carrot Strawberry Smoothie

Prep time: 5 Minutes

Cook time: 5 Minutes

Serves: 2

What you need:

- 1/3 cup Bell Pepper, diced
- 1 cup Carrot Juice, chilled
- 1 cup Mango, diced
- 1 cup Strawberries, unsweetened & frozen

Method:

1. To start with, place strawberries, bell pepper, and mango in the blender pitcher.
2. After that, pulse it a few times.
3. Next, pour the carrot juice into it.
4. Finally, press the 'smoothie' button.

Tip: You can try adding pineapple chunks to it for enhanced flavor.

Per serving: Calorie-66 Kcal Protein-1g Fats- 0g Carbohydrates-14g Sodium-1g Potassium-270mg

Green Smoothie

Prep time: 5 Minutes

Cook time: 5 Minutes

Serves: 3 to 4

What you need:

- 1/4 cup Baby Spinach
- 1/2 cup Ice
- 1/4 cup Kale
- 1/2 cup Pineapple Chunks
- 1/2 cup Coconut Water
- 1/2 cup mango, diced
- 1/2 Banana, diced

Method:

1. Begin by placing all the ingredients needed to make the smoothie in the blender pitcher.
2. Now, press the 'extract' button.
3. Transfer the smoothie into the serving glass.

Per serving: Calories: 207 Carbohydrates: 33 grams Protein: 15 grams Sodium: 73 milligrams Cholesterol: 4 milligrams

Kiwi Smoothie

Prep time: 5 Minutes

Cook time: 5 Minutes

Serves: 3

What you need:

- 1/4 of 1 Avocado, ripe & pitted
- 1/4 cup Ice
- 1/4 cup Coconut Water
- 3/4 cup Kale Leaves
- 1/2 cm Ginger, fresh & peeled
- 2 Kiwis, quartered
- 1 Date pitted & halved
- 1 tsp. Lime Juice

Method:

1. First, place ice, kale leaves, avocado, dates, kiwis, lime juice, ginger, and coconut water in the blender pitcher.
2. Then, press the 'smoothie' button.
3. Finally, transfer to a serving glass and enjoy it.

Per serving: Calories: 268.0 Total Fat: 2.3 g Cholesterol: 40.0 mg Sodium: 141.2 mg Total Carbs: 34.3 g Dietary Fiber: 6.0 g Protein: 27.9 g

Pineapple Kale Smoothie

Prep time: 5 Minutes

Cook time: 5 Minutes

Serves: 3

What you need:

- 3/4 cup Kale leaves
- 1 cup Pineapple, fresh & chopped into chunks
- 1/4 cup Ice
- 3/4 cup Coconut Water
- 1/4 of 1 Avocado, ripe & pitted
- 1/2 of 1 Lime
- 1 Date pitted & halved

Method:

1. For making this bright, tasty smoothie, place ice, kale leaves, avocado, date, coconut water, lime, and pineapple in the blender pitcher.
2. After that, press the 'smoothie' button.
3. Finally, transfer the smoothie to a serving glass and enjoy it.
4. For a richer smoothie, you can try substituting coconut water with light coconut milk.

Per serving: Calories: 266.3 Total Fat: 0.6 g Cholesterol: 0.0 mg Sodium: 34.9 mg Total Carbs: 68.6 g Dietary Fiber: 8.8 g Protein: 4.0 g

Antioxidant Smoothie

Prep time: 5 Minutes

Cook time: 5 Minutes

Serves: 3

What you need:

- 1/2 cup Celery Stalk, halved
- 1/3 cup Watermelon, chopped into chunks
- 1/4 cup Ice
- 1/8 cup Red Cabbage, chopped
- 1/2 cup Blueberries
- 1/2 cup Pomegranate Juice
- 1/2 of 1 Apple, unpeeled & halved

Method:

1. Begin by placing ice, red cabbage, celery stalk, apple, blueberries, and watermelon in the blender pitcher.
2. Now, select the 'smoothie' button.
3. Finally, transfer the smoothie to the serving glass and enjoy it.

Per serving: Calories: 225.3 Total Fat: 9.1 g Cholesterol: 10.0 mg Sodium: 135.5 mg Total Carbs: 29.7 g Dietary Fiber: 7.2 g Protein: 9.1 g

Carrot Beetroot Smoothie

Prep time: 5 Minutes

Cook time: 5 Minutes

Serves: 3

What you need:

- 1/2 of 1 Beet, small & halved
- 3/4 cup Water
- 1/2 cup Ice
- 1 Celery Stalk
- 1/2 of 1 Lemon
- 1/2 of 1 Carrot, halved
- 1/2 cm Ginger, fresh & peeled
- 1/2 of 1 Orange, halved

Method:

1. To start with, place ice, carrot, beet, celery stalk, lemon, ginger, orange, and water in the blender pitcher.
2. Then select the 'smoothie' button.
3. Finally, transfer the smoothie to the serving glass.

Tip: For a more vibrant smoothie, you can try substituting coconut water with light coconut milk.

Per serving: Calories: 169.7 Total Fat: 1.0 g Cholesterol: 0.0 mg Sodium: 112.3 mg Total Carbs: 38.3 g Dietary Fiber: 3.6 g Protein: 3.7 g

Chocolate Avocado Smoothie

Prep time: 5 minutes

Cook time: 0 minute

Serves: 2

What you need:

- 1 cup
- Spinach (fresh or frozen)
- 2 scoops Soy protein isolate (chocolate flavor)
- Two bananas (peeled)
- One small Hass avocado (peeled, stoned)
- ¼ cup Flaxseeds
- 3 cups Water

Optional Toppings:

- Lemon slices Mint leaves

Method:

1. Add all the ingredients to a blender and blend until smooth.
2. Serve with the optional toppings and enjoy!
3. Store the smoothie in an airtight container in the fridge, and consume within two days.
4. Store in the freezer for a maximum of 60 days and thaw at room temperature.

Per serving: Calories: 433 Carbs: 36.1 g Fat: 16.2. g. Protein: 35.6 g. Fiber: 12.9 g. Sugar: 15.8 g.

Gingerbread Smoothie

Prep time: 5 minutes

Cook time: 0 minute

Serves: 2

What you need:

- 2 scoops Soy protein isolate (chocolate flavor)
- Two bananas(peeled)
- One medium Hass avocado (peeled, stoned) 2 tbsp. Chia seeds 2 tbsp.5-spice powder
- 3 cups Water

Optional Toppings:

- Blueberries Shredded coconut Cocoa powder

Method:

1. Add all the ingredients to a blender and blend until smooth.
2. Serve with the optional toppings and enjoy!
3. Store the pudding on airtight container in the fridge, consume within two days.
4. Store in the refrigerator for up to 60 days, then thaw at room temperature.

Per serving: Calories: 392 Carbs: 36.4 g. Fat: 13.4 g. Protein: 31.2 g. Fiber: 10.2 g. Sugar: 14.4 g.

Vegetable Smoothie

Prep time: 3 minutes

Cook time: 0 minutes

Serves: 4

Ingredients

- ½ cucumbers - ½ celery head - 2 cups of spinach (60 gr)
- A handful of mint
- 3 carrots
- ½ handful of parsley
- ¼ pineapple, orange, and lemon
- 2 apples

Method:

1. Place all the ingredients in the blender and mix until a homogeneous mix is obtained
2. Pour into a glass
3. For fast results, drink this smoothie regularly.

Per serving: Calories: 289 Carbohydrate: 58.6g Fat: 6.6g Protein: 5.9g

Natural Protein Shake

Prep time:3 minutes

Cook time: 0 minutes

Serves: 2

What you need:

- ½ bananas - ½ cup of peanut butter (100 gr)
- ½ cup of fat-free milk (125 ml)
- 1 tablespoon of chocolate-flavored whey protein
- From 6 to 8 ice cubes
- Method:
- Pour all the ingredients into a blender
- Blend for a few minutes until the mix becomes homogeneous and consistent
- Pour the smoothie into a glass.

Per serving: Calories: 120 Carbohydrate: 9g Fat: 3 g Protein: 15 g

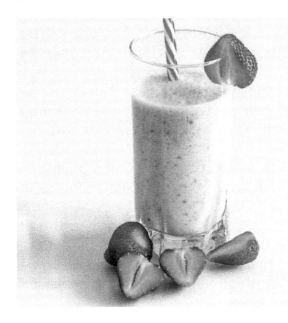

Shrimp Canapé

Prep time: 5 minutes

Cook time: 15 minutes

Serves: 4

What you need:

- 1 rolls of short crust pastry
- Chives
- Tarragon
- 1 cup of prawn tails
- Butter
- Salt
- Brandy
- 1 lemon peel
- 1 cup of mayonnaise
- Pink pepper

Method:

1. Roll out the short crust pastry, sprinkle with a chopped aromatic herb to taste, then use a 7 cm pastry cutter to make the bases for your canapés and prick them.
2. Using an inverted (and lightly greased) muffin pan as a mold, give your molds the shape of exceedingly small tacos, taking care to leave the part with the herbs outside.
3. Bake for 10-15 minutes at 180 ° C in a preheated convection oven, then gently turn out and leave to cool.
4. In the meantime, season the prawn tails with salt and brandy and cook them in a pan with the butter.
5. Assemble the canapés: add 1 shrimp into each brisée base, and then decorate with mayonnaise, lemon peel, and pink pepper.
6. The prawn canapés are ready; you just must serve them and delight your guests.

Per serving: Calories: 180 Carbohydrate: 10g Fat: 2 g Protein: 12 g

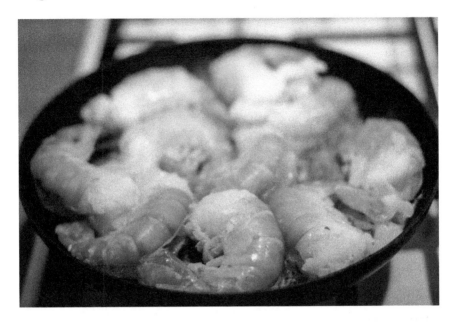

Chocolate Banana Protein Smoothie

Prep time: 5 minutes

Cook time: 0 minutes

Serves: 2

What you need:

•1 frozen banana

•1/3 cup frozen strawberries

•1 cup of silken tofu

•4 Medjool dates, soaked

•2 tablespoons unsweetened cocoa

•1 tablespoon flax meal (optional)

•1 handful kale (optional)

•1 cup milk

Directions

1.Place all the ingredients in your blender and blend until smooth, creamy and a bit frothy.

Per serving: 330 Calories (kcal) 9g Protein 40g Carbs 15g Fat

Med-Style Olives

Prep time: 10 minutes

Cook time: 10 minutes

Serves: 6

What you need:

- One pinch of salt One pinch of black pepper
- 1 ½ tablespoon of coriander seeds
- One tablespoon of extra-virgin olive oil
- One lemon
- 7 oz. of kalamata olives
- 7 oz. of green queen olives

Method:

1. Using a pestle and mortar, finely crush the coriander seeds and set aside.
2. Using a sharp knife, cut long, thin slices of lemon rind and place into a bowl with both the green queen and kalamata olives.
3. Squeeze the juice of one lemon over the top of the olives and add the olive oil.
4. Add the salt, pepper, and coriander seeds, then stir and serve.
5. The longer you allow the olives to rest in the marinade, the more delicious they will taste.

Per serving: Calories: 477; Total Fat: 9g; Carbohydrate: 60g; Dietary Fiber: 3g; Sugar: 5g; Protein: 35g

Roasted Chickpeas

Prep time: 10 minutes

Cook time: 40 minutes

Serves: 6

What you need:

- One pinch of salt
- One pinch of black pepper
- One pinch of garlic powder
- One teaspoon of dried oregano
- Two tablespoons of extra-virgin olive oil
- juice of 1 lemon
- Two teaspoons of red wine vinegar
- 2 15 oz. canned chickpeas

Method:

1. Preheat your oven to 42 5°F and place a sheet of parchment paper onto a baking tray.
2. Drain and rinse the chickpeas, then pour them onto the baking tray. Spread them evenly.
3. Place them in the oven and roast them for 10 minutes.
4. Remove from the oven, give the plate a firm shake, then return the plate to the oven for a further 10 minutes.
5. Once roasted, remove from the oven and set aside. Add the remaining ingredients into a mixing bowl.
6. Combine well, then add the roasted chickpeas.
7. Using a spatula ensures that the chickpeas are evenly coated.
8. Return the chickpeas into the oven and allow to roast for 10 minutes. Remove them from the oven, allow to cool, then serve.
9. Keep checking on the chickpeas while they roast to ensure they do not burn or require longer Cook time.

Per serving: Calories: 323; Total fat: 15.6g; Carbohydrate: 39.5g; Dietary Fiber: 5.3g; Sugar: 11.5g; Protein: 10.4g

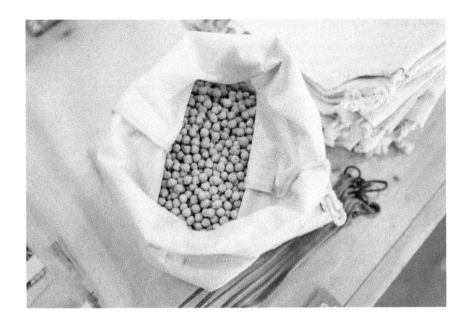

Honey Chili Nuts

Prep time: 10 minutes

Cook time: 30 minutes

Serves: 4

What you need:

- 5oz walnuts
- 5oz pecan nuts
- 2oz softened butter
- 1 tablespoon honey
- ½ bird's-eye chili, very finely chopped and deseeded

Method:

1. Preheat the oven to 180C/360F. Combine the butter, honey, and chili in a bowl, then add the nuts and stir them well.
2. Spread the nuts onto a lined baking sheet and roast them in the oven for 10 minutes, stirring once halfway through.
3. Remove from the oven and allow them to cool before eating.

Per serving: Calories: 65g Fat: 0.5g Fiber: 0.8g Carbs: 4.9g Protein: 2g

Spring Strawberry Kale Salad

Prep time: 5 minutes

Cook time: 15-20 minutes

Serves: 4

Ingredients

- 3 cups baby kale, rinsed and dried
- 10 large strawberries, sliced
- ½ cup honey
- 1/3 cup white wine vinegar
- 1 cup extra virgin olive oil
- 1 tablespoon poppy seeds
- 2 tablespoons pine nuts, toasted
- Salt and pepper to taste

Method:

1. In a large bowl, mix the baby kale with the strawberries.
2. To make the dressing: In a blender, add the honey, vinegar, and oil and blend until smooth.
3. Stir in the poppy seeds and season to taste
4. Pour over the kale and strawberries and toss to coat.

Per serving: Calories: 220cal Carbohydrates: 21g Fat: 15g Protein: 5g

Blackberry Arugula Salad

Prep time: 5 minutes

Cook time: 10 minutes

Serves: 5

Ingredients

- 3 cups baby arugula, rinsed and dried
- 1-pint fresh blackberries
- ¾ cups of crumbled feta cheese
- 1-pint cherry tomatoes, halved
- 1 green onion, sliced
- ¼ cup walnuts, chopped (optional)

To Serve:

- Balsamic reduction, as required

Method:

1. In a large bowl, toss together baby arugula, blackberries, feta cheese, cherry tomatoes, green onion, and walnuts.
2. Drizzle balsamic reduction over plated salads

Per serving: Calories: 270 Fat: 13g Saturated Fat: 2g Carbohydrates: 38g

Apple Walnut Spinach Salad

Prep time: 5 minutes

Cook time: 10 minutes

Serves: 4

Ingredients

- 3 cups baby spinach
- 1 medium apple, chopped
- ¼ Medjool dates, chopped
- ¼ cup walnuts, chopped
- 2 tablespoons extra virgin olive oil
- 1 tablespoon sugar
- 1 tablespoon apple cider vinegar
- ½ teaspoon curry powder
- ¼ teaspoon turmeric
- 1/8 teaspoon chili pepper flakes
- ¼ teaspoon salt

Method:

1. In a large bowl, combine the spinach, apple, dates, and walnuts.
2. To make the dressing: In a jar with a tight-fitting lid, combine the remaining ingredients; shake well.
3. Drizzle over salad and toss to coat.

Per serving: Calories: 166.1 Fat: 11.9g Cholesterol: 5.0g Carbohydrates: 12.6g

Enhanced Waldorf salad

Prep time: 5 minutes

Cook time: 2 hours

Serves: 4

Ingredients

- 4 – 5 stalks celery, sliced
- 1 medium apple, chopped
- ¼ cup walnuts, chopped
- 1 small red onion, diced
- 1 head of red endive, chopped
- 2 teaspoons fresh parsley, finely diced
- 1 tablespoon capers, drained
- 2 teaspoons Lovage or celery leaves, finely diced

For the dressing:

- 1 tablespoon extra-virgin olive oil
- 1 teaspoon balsamic vinegar
- 1 teaspoon Dijon mustard
- Juice of half a lemon

Method:

1. To make the dressing: Whisk together the oil, vinegar, mustard, and lemon juice.
2. Add the remaining salad ingredients to a medium – large-sized salad bowl and toss.
3. Drizzle the dressing over the salad, mix, and serve cold.

Per serving: Calorie: 582Kcal Fat: 103g Fat: 22.2g Protein: 8.2g

Kale Salad with Pepper Jelly Dressing

Prep time: 5 minutes

Cook time: 20 minutes

Serves: 4

Ingredients

- 4 tablespoons mild pepper jelly
- 3 tablespoons olive oil
- ¼ teaspoon salt
- ½ teaspoon Dijon mustard
- 3 cups baby kale leaves
- ½ cup goat cheese, crumbled
- ¼ cup walnuts, chopped

Method:

1. To make the dressing: In a small bowl, whisk together the pepper jelly, olive oil, salt, and mustard.
2. Heat in the microwave for 30 seconds. Let cool.
3. Place the kale in a large bowl and toss with the dressing. Serve topped with goat cheese and sprinkle with walnuts.

Per serving: Calories: 1506.3 Kcal Cholesterol: 25.3mg Carbohydrates: 96.3g

Hot Arugula and Artichoke Salad

Prep time: 5 minutes

Cook time: 10 minutes

Serves: 2

Ingredients

- 1 tablespoon extra-virgin olive oil
- 2 cups baby arugula, washed and dried
- 1 red onion, thinly sliced
- 1 (3/4 cups) jar marinated artichoke hearts, quartered or chopped
- 1 cup feta cheese, crumbled

Method:

1. Preheat oven to 300 degrees F.
2. Drizzle olive oil on a rimmed baking sheet. Spread arugula in a thick layer covering the baking sheet.
3. Arrange onions and artichokes over the spinach and drizzle the marinade from the jar over the entire salad.
4. Sprinkle with the cheese and bake for about 10 minutes, or until the arugula is wilted but NOT crispy.
5. Serve warm.

Per serving: Calories: 281Kcal Fat: 26.g Cholesterol: 126mg Protein: 7g

Spinach and Chicken Salad

Prep time: 5 minutes

Cook time: 30 minutes

Serves: 4

Ingredients

- 2 cups fresh spinach, rinsed and dried
- 4 cooked skinless, boneless chicken breast halves, sliced
- 1 zucchini, halved lengthwise and sliced
- 1 red bell pepper, chopped
- ½ cup black olives
- ¼ cup capers, drained
- ½ cups fontina cheese, frozen and shredded

Method:

1. Place equal portions of spinach onto four salad plates.
2. Arrange chicken, zucchini, bell pepper, and black olives and capers over spinach and top with
3. Cheese.

Per serving: Calories: 120 Fat: 4.9g Cholesterol: 15mg Carbohydrates: 13g

Warm Citrus Chicken Salad

Prep time: 10 minutes

Cook time: 20 minutes

Serves: 4

Ingredients

- 3 cups torn fresh kale
- 2 mandarin oranges, peeled and pulled into individual segments
- ½ cup mushrooms, sliced
- 1 small red onion, sliced
- ½ pound skinless, boneless chicken breast halves - cut into strips
- ¼ cup walnuts, chopped
- 2 tablespoons extra virgin olive oil
- 2 teaspoons cornstarch
- ½ teaspoon ground ginger
- ¼ cup pure orange juice, fresh squeezed is best
- ¼ cup red wine vinegar or apple cider vinegar

Method:

1. The place was torn kale, orange segments, mushrooms, and onion into a large bowl and toss to combine.
2. In a skillet, sauté chicken and walnuts in oil stirring frequently until chicken is no longer pink, a minimum of 10 minutes.
3. In a small bowl, whisk the cornstarch, ginger, orange juice, and vinegar until smooth.
4. Stir into the chicken mixture. Bring to a boil and simmer, continually stirring for 2 minutes or until thickened and bubbly.
5. Serve salads and pour chicken mixture over the top.

Per serving: Calories: 237 Fat: 11.3g Carbohydrates: 9.8g Cholesterol: 101.9mg

Summer Buckwheat Salad

Prep time: 15 minutes

Cook time: 30 minutes

Serves: 4

Ingredients

- ½ cup buckwheat groats
- ¾ cup corn kernels
- 2 medium-sized carrots, diced
- 1 spring onion, diced
- ¼ cucumber, chopped
- 1 red onion, diced
- 10 radishes, chopped
- 3 cups cooked black beans

Method:

1. Using a fine-mesh sieve, rinse the buckwheat under running water
2. Bring to a boil in 1 cup of water, and then reduce to a simmer, covered, for 10 minutes
3. Drain well and chill in the fridge for at least 30 minutes
4. Combine cooled buckwheat and remaining ingredients in a large salad bowl

Per serving: Calories: 128 Fat: 22g Protein: 4g

Greek-Style Shrimp Salad on a Bed of Baby Kale

Prep time: 15 minutes

Cook time: 30 minutes

Serves: 4

Ingredients

- 1-pound raw shrimp (26 to 30), peeled
- ¼ cup extra virgin olive oil plus more, as needed for grilling
- Salt and pepper to taste
- Sugar to taste
- 2 medium tomatoes, diced
- ½ cup feta cheese, crumbled
- ½ cup black olives, sliced
- 1 teaspoon dried oregano
- 4 teaspoons red wine vinegar
- 3 cups of baby kale

Method:

1. Preheat a gas grill or barbeque on high.
2. Thread shrimp onto metal skewers (or bamboo ones that have been soaked in water for 15 minutes).
3. Brush both sides with oil and season with salt, pepper, and sugar, to taste.
4. Grill shrimp until fully cooked and spotty brown, about 2 minutes per side.
5. Meanwhile, in a medium-sized bowl, combine the tomatoes, cheese, olives, oregano, 2 tablespoons. Of the olive oil and 2 teaspoons of the vinegar.
6. When the shrimp is cooked, unthread it carefully and add to bowl. Lightly toss all the ingredients to coat. Set aside.

7. When ready to serve, drizzle remaining oil over kale in a large bowl, tossing to coat. Add remaining vinegar and toss again.
8. Divide kale among 4 large plates. Top each with a portion of the shrimp mixture.

Per serving: Calories: 460 Carbohydrates: 13g Fat: 33g Protein: 30g

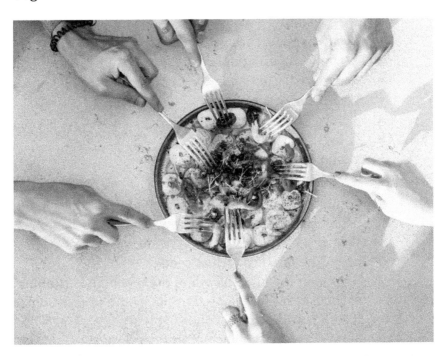

Walnut Herb Pesto

Prep time: 5 minutes

Cook time: 3 Minutes

Serves: 4-6

Ingredients

- 1 cup walnuts
- ¾ cup parsley, chopped
- ¾ cup Lovage, chopped
- ¾ cup basil, chopped
- ½ cup Parmesan, grated
- 3 cloves of garlic, chopped
- ½ teaspoon salt
- ½ cup extra virgin olive oil

Method:

1. Combine all ingredients except olive oil in a food processor and pulse for a few seconds to combine. You may need to scrape down the sides a few times to get the mixture well pureed.
2. Drizzle in the olive oil while the machine is running to incorporate the oil – don't over the process once the oil is added, 30 seconds is plenty
3. Serve with crisped baguette slices or pasta

Per serving: Calories: 31 Fat: 3.1g Carbohydrates: 0.8g

Creamy Lovage Dressing

Prep time: 5 minutes

Cook time: 0 mins

Serves: 2-3

Ingredients

- 1 lemon, juiced
- 1 teaspoon garlic powder
- 1 teaspoon dried onion powder
- 1 teaspoon Dijon mustard
- 1 teaspoon Lovage
- ¼ cup walnuts, soaked
- 1 teaspoon date or maple syrup
- Salt and pepper to taste

Method:

1. Blend the soaked nuts with the date syrup to make walnut butter.
2. Place all ingredients in a small mixing bowl.
3. Whisk well to combine.

Per serving: Calories: 90Kcal Carbohydrates: 6g Fat: 8g Protein:0

Sesame Tofu Salad

Prep time: 12 minutes

Cook time: 30 minutes

Serves: 2

Ingredients

- Cooked tofu – 0.625g (shredded)
- Cucumber – 1 (peel, halve lengthways, deseed with a teaspoon and slice)
- Sesame seeds - 1 tablespoon
- Baby kale - 0.4375 g (roughly chopped)
- Red onion – ½ (shredded finely)
- Pak choi – ½ cup (shredded finely)
- Large handful (20g) parsley, chopped

For the Dressing

- Soy sauce - 2 teaspoon
- Sesame oil - 1 teaspoon
- Extra virgin olive oil - 1 tablespoon
- Juice of 1 lime
- Honey or maple syrup- 1 teaspoon

Method:

1. Toast the sesame seeds in a dry frypan for approx. Two minutes until fragrant and lightly browned. Transfer the seeds to a plate to cool.
2. Mix the lime juice, soy sauce, honey, sesame oil, and olive oil in a small bowl to get your dressing.
3. Place the Pak choi, parsley, red onion, kale, and cucumber in a large bowl. Mix. Add to the bowl of the dressing and mix again.
4. Share the salad into two plates, and then add the shredded tofu on top. Sprinkle over the sesame seeds before you serve.

Per serving: Total Fat: 200 Carbohydrate: 8g Fat: 12g Protein: 20g

Turmeric Extract Poultry & Kale Salad with Honey Lime Dressing

Prep time: 10 minutes

Cook time: 30 minutes

Serves: 2

What you need:

For the chicken:

- 1 teaspoon coconut oil
- 1/2 tool brown onion, diced
- 250-300 g/ 9 oz. hens mince or diced up her thighs
- 1 large garlic clove, finely diced
- 1 tsp turmeric powder
- 1teaspoon lime passion
- Juice of 1/2 lime
- 1/2 tsp salt + pepper

For the salad:

- 6 broccoli stalks or broccoli florets
- 2 tablespoons pumpkin seeds (pepitas).
- 3 huge kale leaves, stems eliminated and chopped.
- 1/2 avocado, sliced.
- Handful of fresh coriander leaves, chopped.
- Handful of fresh parsley leaves, sliced.

For the clothing:

- 3 tablespoons lime juice.
- 1 small garlic clove, finely grated.
- 3 tbsps. Extra-virgin olive oil (I made use of 1 tbsp. avocado oil and * 2 tbsps. EVO).
- 1 tsp raw honey.
- 1/2 tsp wholegrain or Dijon mustard.
- 1/2 teaspoon sea salt and pepper.

Method:

1. Warm the ghee or coconut oil in a small frying pan over medium-high warmth. Include the onion and sauté on medium heat for 4-5 mins, until golden. Include the hen dice as well as garlic and mix for 2-3 minutes over medium-high warm, breaking it apart.
2. Add the turmeric extract, lime enthusiasm, lime juice, salt, and pepper, and cook, frequently mixing, for a further 3-4 mins. Establish the cooked dice apart.
3. While the poultry is cooking, bring a small saucepan of water to steam. Add the broccolini and prepare for 2 mins. Wash under cold water as well as cut into 3-4 pieces each.
4. Include the pumpkin seeds to the frying pan from the poultry and toast over tool warmth for 2 mins, often mixing to avoid burning season with a little salt. Allot. Raw pumpkin seeds are too high to make use of.
5. The area sliced Kale in a salad bowl as well as pour over the clothing. Utilizing your hands, throw as well as massage the Kale with the dress. This will undoubtedly soften the Kale, kind of like what citrus juice does to fish or beef carpaccio-- it 'cooks' it slightly.
6. Finally toss via the prepared hen, broccolini, fresh, natural herbs, pumpkin seeds, and avocado pieces.

Per serving: Calories: 368 Carbohydrate: 30.3g Protein 6.7g Fat: 27.6g

Buckwheat Pasta with Chicken Kale & Miso Dressing

Prep time: 15 minutes

Cook time: 15 minutes

Serves: 2

What you need:

For the noodles:

- 2-3 handfuls of kale leaves (eliminated from the stem as well as approximately cut).
- 150 g/ 5 oz. 100% buckwheat noodles.
- 3-4 shiitake mushrooms cut.
- 1 tsp coconut oil or ghee.
- 1 brownish onion carefully diced.
- 1 medium free-range chicken breast cut or diced.
- 1 long red chili very finely sliced (seeds in or out depending upon how warm you like it).
- 2 big garlic cloves finely diced.
- 2-3 tablespoons Tamari sauce (gluten-free soy sauce).

For the miso dressing:

- 1 1/2 tbsp. fresh, natural miso.
- 1 tbsp. Tamari sauce.
- 1 tbsp. extra-virgin olive oil.
- 1 tbsp. lemon or lime juice.
- 1 teaspoon sesame oil (optional).

Method:

1. Bring a tool saucepan of water to steam. Include the Kale as well as cook for 1 min, up until a little wilted. Remove as well as reserve yet schedule the water and bring it back to the boil. Add the soba noodles and chef according to the bundle guidelines

(typically about 5 mins). Rinse under cold water and allotted.

2. Then pan fry the mushrooms in coconut oil (concerning a tsp) for 2-3 minutes until gently browned on each side. Sprinkle with sea salt and allotted.

3. In the very same frypan, warmth a lot more coconut oil or ghee over medium-high warm. Sauté onion and chili for 2-3 mins and then add the poultry pieces. Cook 5 mins over medium warmth, stirring a couple of times, after that, add the garlic, tamari sauce, and a little splash of water. Cook for a more 2-3 mins, often mixing till hen is cooked via.

4. Lastly, include the kale and soba noodles and toss with the poultry to warm up.

5. Mix the dressing and drizzle over the noodles right at the end of cooking; this way, you will certainly maintain all those beneficial probiotics in the miso to life as well as energetic.

Per serving: Calories: 260 Carbohydrate: 35.3g Protein 15g Cholesterol: 50g Fat: 27.6g

Sirtfood Lentil Super Salad

Prep time: 10 minutes

Cook time: 0 minutes

Serves: 1

What you need:

- 20 g red onion, sliced
- 1 tbsp. extra virgin olive oil
- 1 large Medjool date, chopped
- 1 tbsp. capers
- ¼ cup rocket
- 2 avocados, peeled, stoned and sliced
- 100 g lentils
- ¼ cup chicory leaves
- 2 tbsp. chopped walnuts
- 1 tbsp. fresh lemon juice
- ¼ cup chopped parsley
- ¼ cup chopped celery leaves

Method:

1. Arrange salad leaves in a large bowl or a plate; mix the remaining ingredients well and serve over the salad leaves.

Per serving: Calories: 456 Carbs: 54 Protein: 27 Fat: 11

Sirty Fruit Salad

Prep time: 10 minutes

Cook time: 0 minutes

Serves: 1

What you need:

- 10 blueberries
- 10 red seedless grapes
- ½ cup brewed green tea
- 1 apple, cored, chopped
- 1 tsp. honey
- 1 orange, chopped
- 2 tbsp. fresh lemon juice

Method:

1. Add honey into a cup of green tea and stir until dissolved; add orange juice and set aside to cool.
2. Place the chopped orange in a bowl and add grapes, apple and blueberries; pour over the tea and let steep for at least 5 minutes before serving.

Per serving: Calories per serving: 362.47 kcal Carbs per serving: 25.39 g Fats per serving: 9.34 g Proteins per serving: 5.28 g Fiber per serving: 2.86 g Sodium per serving: 9.

Superfood Cleansing Salad with Citrus Dressing

Prep time: 15 minutes

Cook time: 0 minutes

Serves: 4

What you need:

- 2 cups red cabbage, chopped
- 2 cups kale, chopped
- 1 head cauliflower, roughly chopped
- 1 red onion
- 2 cups baby carrots
- 1/3 cup fresh cilantro, chopped
- 1/3 cup sunflower seeds
- 1/2 cup raisins
- 1/2 cup raw hemp hearts

Citrus Dressing:

- 2 tablespoons fresh lime juice
- 2 tablespoons fresh lemon juice
- 1/3 cup apple cider vinegar
- 1/2 avocado
- 2 cloves garlic
- 1/2 tablespoon fresh cilantro
- 1/2 tablespoon minced ginger
- 1/2 tablespoon raw honey
- 1/2 teaspoon sea salt
- 1/4 teaspoon pepper

Directions

1. Combine cabbage, kale, cauliflower, onion, carrots and cilantro in a food processor; shred.
2. Transfer the shredded veggies to a large bowl and fold in sunflower seeds, hemp hearts and raisins.
3. Combine all dressing ingredients in a blender and blend until very smooth.
4. Serve the salad in salad bowls drizzled with the citrus dressing. Enjoy!

Per serving: Calories 91 kcal Fat 8.3 g Cholesterol 0 mg Carbohydrate 12.5 g Fat 0.5 g Protein 4. 4 g Sodium 810 mg

Apple Pancakes with Blackcurrant Compote

Prep time: 10 minutes

Cook time: 15 minutes

Serves: 4

What you need:

- 75g porridge oats sirtfood plans
- 125g plain flour
- 1 tsp preparing powder
- 2 tbsp caster sugar
- Touch of salt
- Two apples, stripped, cored, and cut into little pieces
- 300ml semi-skimmed milk
- Two egg whites
- 2 tsp light olive oil
- For the compote:
- 120g blackcurrants washed and stalks expelled
- 2 tbsp caster sugar
- 3 tbsp water

Method:

1. First, make the compote. Spot the blackcurrants, sugar, and water in a little container. Raise to a stew and cook for 10-15 minutes.
2. Place the oats, flour, heating powder, caster sugar and salt in a large bowl and blend well. Mix in the apple and afterwards speed in the milk a little at once until you have a smooth blend. Whisk the egg whites to hardened pinnacles and afterwards overlay into the hotcake player. Move the player to a container.
3. Warm 1/2 tsp oil in a skillet on a medium-high warmth and pour in around one-fourth of the player. Cook on the two sides until brilliant darker. Expel and rehash to make four hotcakes.

4. Serve the flapjacks with the blackcurrant compote showered over.

Per serving: calories 441, protein 32g, fat 5g, carbohydrates 72g, sodium 7mg.

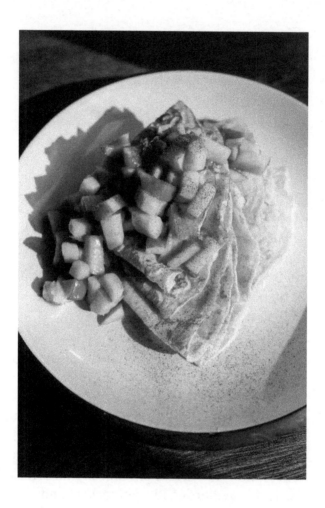

Superfoods Raw Vegan Cookies

Prep time: 10 minutes

Cook time: 30 minutes

Serves: 4

What you need:

- ½ cup of coconut milk
- ½ cup of cocoa powder
- ½ cup of coconut oil
- ½ cup raw honey
- 2 cups finely shredded coconut
- 1 cup large flake coconut
- 2 tsp of ground vanilla bean
- ½ cup chopped almonds or chia seeds (optional)
- ½ cup almond butter (optional)

Method:

1. Combine the coconut milk, cocoa powder, and coconut oil in a saucepan.
2. I think that it still counts as a raw dessert if you must warm up the coconut milk and coconut oil.
3. So, warm up the mixture over medium heat because we want the coconut oil to melt and become liquid.

Nutrients: Calories: 209 Cal Fat: 11 g

Raw Vegan Walnuts Pie Crust & Raw Brownies

Prep time: 10 minutes

Cook time: 30 minutes

Serves: 4

What you need:

- 1½ cups walnuts
- 1 cup pitted dates
- 1½ tsp ground vanilla bean
- 2 tsp chia seeds
- 1/3 cup unsweetened cocoa powder
- Topping for raw brownies:
- 1/3 cup almond butter

Method:

1. Add walnuts to a food processor or blender.
2. Mix until finely ground.
3. Add the vanilla, dates, and cocoa powder to the blender.
4. Mix well and optionally add a couple of drops of water at a time to make the mixture stick together.
5. This is an essential raw walnuts pie crust recipe.
6. You can use almonds or cashews as well.
7. If you need a pie crust, then spread it thinly in a 9-inch disc and add the filling.
8. If you want to make raw brownies, then transfer the mixture into a small dish and top with almond butter.

Per serving: Calories per serving: 293 Fat: 6.3g Protein: 4. 8g Carbs: 36g Sodium: 0mg Sugars: 1.4g Fiber: 5.1g

Herby French Fries with Herbs and Avocado Dip

Prep time: 20 minutes

Cook time: 35 minutes

Serves: 2

What you need:

For the Fries:

- 1/2 pieces Celery
- 150 g Sweet potato
- 1 teaspoon dried oregano
- 1 / 2 teaspoon Dried basil
- 1/2 teaspoon Celtic sea salt
- 1 teaspoon Black pepper
- 1 1/2 tablespoon Coconut oil (melted)
- Baking paper sheet
- For the avocado dip
- 1-piece Avocado
- 4 tablespoons Olive oil
- 1 tablespoon Mustard
- 1 teaspoon Apple cider vinegar
- 1 tablespoon Honey
- 2 cloves Garlic (pressed)
- 1 teaspoon dried oregano

Method:

1. Preheat the oven to 205 ° C.
2. Peel the celery and sweet potatoes.
3. Cut the celery and sweet potatoes into (thin) French fries.
4. Place the French fries in a large bowl and mix with the coconut oil and herbs.
5. Shake the bowl a few times so that the fries are covered with a layer of the oil and herb mixture.

6. Place the chips in a layer on a baking sheet lined with baking paper or on a grill rack.
7. Bake for 25-35 minutes (turn over after half the time) until they have a nice golden-brown color and are crispy.
8. For the avocado dip
9. Puree all ingredients evenly with a hand blender or blender.

Per serving: Calories: 146 Cal Fat: 12 g Carbs: 87.98 g Protein: 14.51 g Fiber: 35.8 g

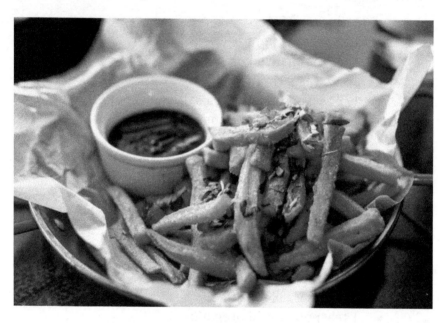

Salad with Bacon, Cranberries and Apple

Prep time: 10 minutes

Cook time: 5 minutes

Serves: 2

What you need:
- 1 hand Arugula
- 4 slices Bacon
- 1/2 pieces Apple
- 2 tablespoon Dried cranberries
- 1/2 pieces Red onion
- 1/2 pieces Red bell pepper
- 1 hand Walnuts

Dressing:
- 1 teaspoon Mustard yellow
- 1 teaspoon Honey
- 3 tablespoon Olive oil

Method:
1. Warm a pan over medium heat and fry the bacon until crispy.
2. Place the bacon on a piece of kitchen roll so that the excess fat is absorbed.
3. Cut half the red onion into thin rings. Cut the bell pepper into small cubes.
4. Cut the apple into four pieces and remove the core. Then cut into thin wedges.
5. Drizzle some lemon juice on the apple wedges so that they do not change color.
6. Roughly chop walnuts.
7. Combine the ingredients for the dressing in a bowl. Season with salt and pepper.
8. Spread the lettuce on a plate / your lunch box and season with red pepper, red onions, apple wedges and walnuts.

9. Sprinkle the bacon over the salad and divide the cranberries.
10. Drizzle the dressing over the salad according to taste.

Per serving: Calories: 98 Cal Fat: 82.05 g Carbs: 50.94 g Protein: 15.82 g Fiber: 7.1 g

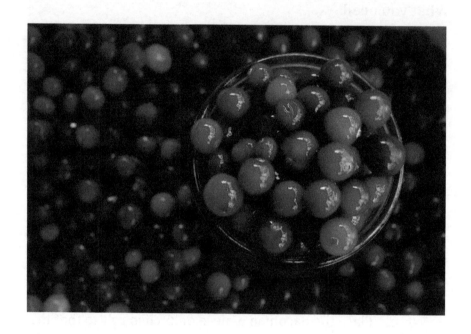

Strawberry Popsicles with Chocolate Dip

Prep time: 20 minutes

Cook time: 10 minutes plus freezing time

Serves: 5

What you need:

- 125 g Strawberries
- 80 ml Water
- 100 g Pure chocolate (> 70% cocoa)

Method:

1. Wash the strawberries and slice them into pieces. Puree the strawberries with the water.
2. If the mixture is not pourable, add some extra water.
3. Pour the mixture into the popsicle mold and put it in a skewer.
4. Place the molds in the freezer so the popsicles can freeze hard.
5. Once the popsicles are frozen hard, you can melt the chocolate in a water bath.
6. Dip the popsicles in the melted chocolate mixture.

Per serving: Calories: 319 Cal Fat: 1.51 g Carbs: 74.7 g Protein: 2.94 g Fiber: 5.1 g

Hawaii Salad

Prep time: 10 minutes

Cook time: 0 minutes

Serves: 2 - 3

What you need:

- 1 hand Arugula
- 1/2 pieces Red onion
- 1-piece Winter carrot
- 2 pieces Pineapple slices
- 80 g Diced ham
- 1 pinch Salt
- 1 pinch Black pepper

Method:

1. Slice the red onion into thin half rings.
2. Remove the peel and hard core from the pineapple and cut the pulp into thin pieces.
3. Clean the carrot and use a spiralizer to make strings.
4. Mix rocket and carrot in a bowl. Spread this over a plate / lunch box.
5. Spread the red onion, pineapple and diced ham over the rocket.
6. Sprinkle the olive oil and balsamic vinegar on the salad to your taste.
7. Season with salt and pepper.

Per serving: Calories: 198 Cal Fat: 2.99 g Carbs: 29.59 g Protein: 15.47 g Fiber: 4 g

Rainbow Salad

Prep time: 10 minutes

Cook time: 0 minutes

Serves: 2 - 3

What you need:

- 1 hand Salad
- 1/2 pieces Avocado
- 1-piece Egg
- 1/4 pieces green peppers
- 1/4 pieces Red bell pepper
- 2 pieces Tomato
- 1/2 pieces Red onion
- 4 tablespoons Carrot (grated)

Method:

1. Boil the egg as you like. (soft / hard / in between)
2. Take away the seeds from the peppers and cut the peppers into thin strips.
3. Cut the tomatoes into small cubes.
4. Slice the red onion into thin half rings.
5. Cut the avocado into thin slices.
6. Cool the egg under running water, peel and cut into slices. Place the salad on a plate / in your lunch box and distribute all the vegetables in colorful rows.
7. If you feel artistic, you can sort the colors from light to dark. Drizzle the vegetables with olive oil and white wine vinegar. Season with salt and pepper.

Per serving: Calories: 158 Cal Fat: 39.7 g Carbs: 49.64 g Protein: 17.16 g Fiber: 20.9 g

Strawberry and Coconut Ice Cream

Prep time: 15 minutes

Cook time: 10 minutes plus freezing time

Serves: 10

What you need:

- 400 ml Coconut milk (can)
- 1 hand Strawberries
- 1/2 pieces Lime
- 3 tablespoons Honey

Method:

1. Clean the strawberries and cut them into large pieces.
2. Grate the lime, 1 teaspoon of lime peel is required. Squeeze the lime.
3. Put all ingredients in a blender and puree everything evenly.
4. Pour the mixture into a bowl and put it in the freezer for 1 hour.
5. Take out the mix out of the freezer and put it in the blender. Mix them well again.
6. Put the mixture back into the bowl and freeze it until it is hard.
7. Before serving; Take it out of the freezer about 10 minutes before scooping out the balls.

Per serving: Calories: 206 Cal Fat: 0.07 g Carbs: 56.54 g Protein: 24 g Fiber: 0.45 g

Coffee Ice Cream

Prep time: 15 minutes

Cook time: 10 minutes plus freezing time

Serves: 10

What you need:
- 180 ml Coffee
- 8 pieces Medjoul dates
- 400 ml Coconut milk (can)
- 1 teaspoon Vanilla extract

Method:
1. See to it that the coffee has cooled down before using it.
2. Cut the dates into rough pieces.
3. Place the dates and coffee in a food processor and mix to an even mass.
4. Add coconut milk and vanilla and puree evenly.
5. Pour the mixture in a bowl and put in the freezer for 1 hour.
6. Take out the mix out of the freezer and scoop it into the blender.
7. Pour it back into the bowl and freeze it until it's hard.
8. When serving; Take it out of the freezer a few minutes before scooping ice cream balls with a spoon.

Per serving: Calories: 172 Cal Fat: 0.22 g Carbs: 43.15 g Protein: 1.39 g Fiber: 4.5 g

Banana Dessert

Prep time: 15 minutes

Cook time: 10 minutes

Serves: 2 - 3

What you need:

- 2 pieces Banana (ripe)
- 2 tablespoons Pure chocolate (> 70% cocoa)
- 2 tablespoons Almond leaves

Method:

1. Chop the chocolate finely, cut the banana lengthwise, but not completely, as the banana must serve as a casing for the chocolate.
2. Slightly slide on the banana, spread the finely chopped chocolate and almonds over the bananas.
3. Fold a kind of boat out of the aluminum foil that supports the banana well, with the cut in the banana facing up.
4. Place the two packets on the grill and grill them for about 4 minutes until the skin is dark.

Per serving: Calories: 232 Cal Fat: 2.08 g Carbs: 51.3 g Protein: 2.15 g Fiber: 2.3 g

Salad with Roasted Carrots

Prep time: 10 minutes

Cook time: 5 minutes

Serves: 2 - 3

What you need:

- 1 hand mixed salad
- 500 g Carrot
- 1 piece Orange
- 100 g Pecans
- 1/2 teaspoon dried thyme
- 1 tablespoon Honey
- 1 tablespoon Olive oil
- 1 pinch Salt
- 1 pinch Black pepper

Method:

1. Peel the carrots and cut the green. Cut them in half lengthways.
2. Cook the carrots al dente for 5 minutes and drain well.
3. Peel the orange and cut it into pieces.
4. Roughly chop the pecans and briefly fry them in a pan without oil.
5. Cut the spring onions into thin rings.
6. Place the carrots in a bowl with 1 tablespoon of olive oil, a pinch of salt and pepper and the thyme.
7. Roast the carrots briefly on the grill or in a grill pan. Until they have nice grill marks.
8. Mix the salad with carrots and honey and put on a plate.
9. Spread the orange slices and pecans over the salad.

Per serving: Calories: 108 Cal Fat: 86.68 g Carbs: 79.26 g Protein: 13.93 g Fiber: 23.8 g

Salmon with Capers and Lemon

Prep time: 10 minutes

Cook time: 15 minutes

Serves: 2 - 3

What you need:

- 2 pieces Salmon fillet
- 1 tablespoon Coconut oil
- 2 tablespoon Capers

Method:

1. Cut the lemon into thin slices.
2. Take an aluminum tray or piece of aluminum foil that is folded in half.
3. First lay out 4 slices of lemon and spread the capers on them.
4. Place the salmon on the capers. Then put a lemon wedge on the salmon.
5. Fry the salmon on the grill (with aluminum dish / foil).
6. Season with salt and pepper just before serving.

Per serving: Calories: 121 Cal Fat: 13.75 g Carbs: 0.84 g Protein: 0.41 g Fiber: 0.6 g

Pine and Sunflower Seed Rolls

Prep time: 20 minutes

Cook time: 35 minutes

Serves: 12

What you need:

- 120 g Tapioca flour
- 1 teaspoon Celtic sea salt
- 4 tablespoon Coconut flour
- 120 ml Olive oil
- 120 ml Water (warm)
- 1-piece Egg (beaten)
- 150 g Pine nuts (roasted)
- 150 g Sunflower seeds (roasted)
- Baking paper sheet

Method:

1. Preheat the oven to 160 ° C.
2. Put the pine nuts and sunflower seeds in a small bowl and set aside.
3. Mix the tapioca with the salt and tablespoons of coconut flour in a large bowl. Pour the olive oil and warm water into the mixture.
4. Add the egg and mix until you get an even batter. Add 1 tablespoon of coconut flour at a time until it has the desired consistency if the dough is too thin.
5. Wait a few minutes between each addition of the flour so that it can absorb the moisture. The dough should be soft and sticky.
6. With a wet tablespoon, take tablespoons of batter to make a roll. Put some tapioca flour on your hands so the dough doesn't stick. Fold the dough with your fingertips instead of rolling it in your palms.
7. Place the roll in the bowl of pine nuts and sunflower seeds and roll it around until covered. Line a baking sheet with parchment paper. Place the buns on the

baking sheet. Cook in the preheated oven for 35 minutes and serve warm.

Per serving: Calories: 245 Cal Fat: 189.53 g Carbs: 159.26 g Protein: 61.33 g Fiber: 20.2 g

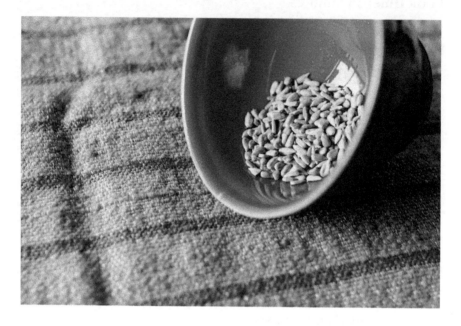

Lightning Source UK Ltd.
Milton Keynes UK
UKHW020658240521
384264UK00005B/150